DASH Diet

For Beginners

Lower Your Blood Pressure For Healthy Weight Loss

Keith Alexander

Disclaimer

The information contained in this book is strictly for educational purpose only. The content of this book is the sole expression and opinion of its author and not necessarily that of the publisher. It is not intended to cure, treat, and diagnose any kind of disease or medical condition. It is sold with the understanding that the publisher is not rendering any type of medical, psychological, legal, or any other kind of professional advice. You should seek the services of a competent professional before applying concepts in this book. Neither the publisher nor the individual author(s) shall be liable for any physical, psychological, emotional, financial, or commercial damages, directly or indirectly by the use of this material, which is provided "as is", and without warranties. Therefore, if you wish to apply ideas contained in this book, you are taking full responsibility for your actions.

Table of Contents

Introduction

Blood pressure, the risk of heart diseases, diabetes, stroke, and weight loss are arguably some of the most discussed issues in the society today. The contribution of diet to all these problems is evident in as much as exercise and other interventions are commonly cited. You are what you eat and your body responds to the nutrients that you take in to your system.

DASH diet is an excellent choice for people who want to lose weight or eat healthy as a measure to safeguard their bodies against infections. DASH diets open up lots of possibilities without hard-to-follow rules, gimmicks or any unreasonable restrictions. As opposed to other diet plans which impose stringent measures and get you stuck in diet doldrums, DASH diet makes you full of energy and enhances your satisfaction.

DASH diet is nutritionally sound, endorsed and approved by the health community and based on extensive scientific experiments. It was chosen by the US News and World Report as a number one diet in the Best Diets for Healthy Eating, Best Diets Overall and Best Diabetes Diets categories. It is not a crash or fad diet but rather a medically developed plan that helps in improving your overall health.

The most interesting thing with DASH diet and certainly the reason behind its popularity is the manner in which it addresses health issues as a matter of priority. Scientific research including laboratory experiments has shown that this diet has a significant impact on cholesterol levels, high blood pressure and kidney functions. Being an excellent weight loss plan, DASH diet has been found to have a beneficial impact on metabolic syndrome, type II diabetes, heart diseases as well as other obesity-related complications.

This book contains everything you need to know to succeed in planning and executing your DASH diet plans. In it, you will find recipes, meal plans and a fitness program. Every plan included can be customized to meet your unique individual requirements.

1: Understanding the DASH Diet

As early as the 1970s, the problem of high blood pressure in the United States had already become rampant. This forced the National Institutes of Health in 1992 to provide funds for research activities aimed at finding a lasting dietary solution to hypertension. The ultimate goal was to come up with dietary approaches to stop hypertension (DASH).

The research was conducted by the National Heart, Lung and Blood Institute through the assistance of five medical research institutions in the United States. These institutions included Duke University Medical Center, Brigham and Women's Hospital, Johns Hopkins University, Pennington Biomedical Research Center and Kaiser Permanente Center for Health Research.

Working in collaboration with one another, these facilities undertook what is considered to be one of the most extensive and exhaustive researches to this day as far as nutrition solutions for hypertension are concerned.

Through randomized control trials, the teams of nutritionists, nurses, doctors, and statisticians worked tirelessly between their institutions. Each of the five facilities picked its own group of participants so as to ensure the findings were not biased. According to the research documentation, more than 8,000 people deliberately went through the screening process under the guidance of the researchers. According to the research requirements, two thirds of the sports were supposed to be filled by participants who were at a high risk of hypertension.

Three diets were used at each facility to test the effect they had on blood pressure. The first diet which was a control diet had a typical resemblance to the standard American diet. It was characterized by low levels of calcium, magnesium, potassium and fiber. The level of fat and protein was also modeled after the average American diet. The factor that was altered in this diet was the level of sodium which was made lower at 1500 mg compared to the average diet. The purpose of this alteration was to represent doctor's recommendations to lower the level of sodium intake so as to subsequently lower blood pressure.

The second diet was similar in composition to the control diet but it had more vegetables and fruits as well as fewer snacks. Its fiber content was also higher than the control diet.

The third and last diet which was the DASH diet had lots of vegetables, fruits, lean protein and low fat dairy. Saturated fats and the overall fat intake were also at their lowest levels. The DASH diet was formulated based on research that revealed the positive impact certain minerals and fiber had on high blood pressure.

Participants in the second and third diets had a sodium intake of 3000 mg daily which represents the average intake of sodium by Americans. The main reason for holding the sodium intake at the normal level was to see whether nutritional changes had a positive impact on hypertension without the need to lower sodium intake.

For purposes of comparisons, two DASH trials were undertaken. The first trial ran from August 1993 all the way to July 1997. The second trial also known as the DASH sodium trial was conducted from September 1997 to November 1999. In the course of each of these trials, the groups were placed on control diet for 3 weeks during which their blood pressure, symptoms and urine were closely monitored. There was a clear difference between the first study and the second one.

The results of the first study revealed that the control diet which had lower sodium levels was very effective in lowering blood pressure. The DASH diet was also effective but to a lesser degree.

This made the DASH diet to be redesigned and to include a lower sodium intake to give it the same property as the control diet while retaining everything else as it was in the initial study. This is the reason why the new diet was referred to as the DASH-sodium diet.

By the end of the second research study, the results showed the control diet as being effective in reducing blood pressure but when compared to the DASH-sodium diet, the effect of the control diet was minimal. This led the researchers to conclude that the DASH diet was the best and more superior in lowering blood pressure. It was high in fiber, contained plenty of vegetables and fresh fruits, low fat dairy, and lean protein.

The observation of the effectiveness of the Dash-sodium diet was reported across all the five research facilities. With a reduced sodium intake of 1500 mg per day, the corresponding responding in blood pressure was 8.9/4.5 mm Hg. These results were recorded just after 30 days on DASH–sodium diet.

The studies described above combined with additional research which came later on showed that the DASH diet is effective in reducing hypertension, body fat, and cholesterol. This was observed to be occasioned by the low sugar intake. Reduced sugar in diets helps in improving insulin sensitivity. Once the body responds more to insulin, it initiates an internal process that increases the disposal or use of stored belly fat.

The findings reported above are the reason why DASH diet is recommended by most medical organizations including the American Heart Association, and the American Medical Association among many others.

DASH Diet Endorsements and Support

DASH diet is endorsed by a number of renowned organizations that include the National Heart, Lung and Blood Institute, 2010 Dietary Guidelines for Americans, Mayo Clinic, 2011 American Heart Association Treatment Guidelines for Women, and The Guidelines for treatment for High Blood Pressure.

The reasons why the above institutions have endorsed and thrown their weight behind a DASH diet is because of the positive effects the diet has on health. Some of the benefits of DASH diet include:

- Lowering the intake of cholesterol and saturated fats which reduces the risk of arterial disease and heart disease.

- Enhancing the intake of healthy fats including Omega 3's which is scientifically known to boost heart health and aid in the loss of abdominal fat. The combination of all this is a reduction in the risk of type II diabetes and metabolic syndromes.

- Lowering high blood pressure which in turn reduces the risk of stroke and heart attack.

The Dietary Guidelines for Americans advise everyone including the elderly and children to participate in the DASH diet eating plan. As a matter of fact, DASH diet formed the basis for the United States Department of Agriculture (USDA) to generate MyPlate dietary guidelines.

2: A Comprehensive Overview of the DASH Diet Plan

The mode through which the DASH diet health plan operates is based on a number of principles. Some of these principles include:

Reduction of Sodium Intake

This step in DASH diet is aimed at lowering hypertension. It is achieved through a standard DASH diet plan which contains up to 2300 mg of sodium intake per day. There is also a low sodium version that allows you to take in up to 1500 mg of sodium in a day. The typical American diet allows up to 3500 mg of sodium in a day and this explains the rampant cases of hypertension.

Increase in Fiber Intake

This works to reduce blood pressure, aid in weight loss and moderate blood sugar levels. Compared to what people are used to eating, the DASH diet provides plenty of vegetables and fresh fruits as well as a wide selection of healthy whole grains.

Reduction in Trans Fat and Saturated Fat

This has a direct effect in enhancing heart health, raising HDL cholesterol, lowering LDL cholesterol, decrease risks of heart disease, metabolic syndrome and diabetes as well as aiding in weight loss. Trans fat comes from fried and processed foods. Usually, these fats are absent in DASH diet because the foods incorporated are low in saturated fats such as seafood, lean meat and low fat dairy.

Increase in Healthy Fats

DASH diet includes foods such as fish, avocado, nuts and seeds which are rich in Omega 3.

Limits Caffeine and Alcohol

These two substances are notorious as far as high blood pressure is concerned. Caffeine being a stimulant causes the heart to beat faster and hence pump large volumes of blood through the vessels which increases vascular pressure.

Monitoring of Mineral Levels

Minerals such as magnesium and potassium are very good in aiding several body functions. If their levels fall below the threshold, they may contribute negatively to blood pressure. By encouraging consumption of a variety of foods which contain minerals such as legumes, bananas, and leafy green vegetables, DASH diet boosts the mineral levels in the body.

Reduction in Risk of Type II Diabetes

Lowering of abdominal fat which is a leading indicator of both type II diabetes and metabolic syndrome, the DASH diet reduces the risk and exposure to these complications. As a matter fact, the DASH diet health plan advocates for a reduction in the intake of sugary foods to no more than 5 per week.

A close examination of the DASH diet shows flexibility not only in sodium intake but also in overall caloric intake. It gives you the flexibility to choose several menu plans which allow either 1500 mg of sodium or 2300 mg of sodium per day. People suffering from high blood pressure or at a high risk of hypertension are advised to settle for the lower intake of sodium. Depending on your caloric needs, you can choose different servings of particular food groups.

1200 Calorie Demand

Individuals with caloric needs of 1200 should take 4 to 5 servings of grains, 3 to 4 servings of vegetables, 3 to 4 servings of fruits, 2 to 3 servings of low fat or fat free dairy products, 3 or less servings of poultry lean meat and fish, 3 servings per week for nuts, legumes and seeds. For fats and oils, only one serving is recommended while for sweets and added sugars, 3 servings or less are recommended per week. The maximum sodium limit for individuals with 1200 caloric demand is 2300 mg per day.

2000 Calorie Demand

Where the calorie demand is 2000, the grain servings should be 6 to 8, vegetables servings at 4 to 5, fruits at 4 to 5 while fat free or low fat dairy products at 2 to 3 servings. When it comes to lean meat, fish and poultry, 6 or fewer servings are recommended. Legumes, seeds and nuts should be between 4 to 5 servings per week, fats and oils at 2 to 3 servings while sweets and added sugars should be maintained at 5 or less servings per week. The maximum sodium limit for this category is 2300 mg per day.

3100 Calorie Demand

This group of individuals is said to be among the most active. As such, they need more energy but at the same time must not comprise on their health status. In the grains food group, the servings should be 12 to 13 while the servings for vegetables and fruits should be maintained at 6 for both food groups.

Low fat dairy products intake should be maintained at 3 to 4 servings, poultry, fish and lean meats at 6 to 9 servings; legumes, seeds and nuts at 1 serving while fats and oils which are among the major contributors of the much needed energy should be maintained at 4 servings. Sweets and added sugars should either be equal to or less than 2 servings. Just like in the above groups, the sodium intake should also be at 2300 mg per day.

Whole grains are usually recommended because they provide an excellent source of nutrients and fiber. Individuals with lactose intolerance can try lactose reduced milk, lactose free milk or lactase enzyme pills combined with dairy products. Fat content changes the serving quantity for oils and fats. For instance, one tablespoon of regular salad dressing is equivalent to one serving; one tablespoon low fat dressing is equivalent to one half serving while one tablespoon fat free dressing is equivalent to zero servings.

3: How the DASH Diet Affects Your Health

Contrary to most diet plans which focus on weight loss, the DASH diet was created to reduce high blood pressure and subsequently prevent the risk posed by heart diseases and stroke. There is so much to learn on how the diet works to improve your health.

DASH Diet and Hypertension

DASH diet plan has been shown to have a direct and significant on high blood pressure. It combines specific nutrients with a low sodium intake which produce positive results in lowering hypertension. According to the Mayo Clinic, following a DASH diet can enhance blood pressure reduction in a matter of weeks.

Your ethnicity, lifestyle, and weight can put you at a high risk of developing hypertension. For instance, African Americans are at a higher risk in developing high blood pressure same to those who smoke and take high quantities of sodium. The DASH diet is recommended by nutritionists and dieticians for reducing your risk.

DASH Diet and Type II Diabetes

According to the US News & World Report, DASH diet is the best for combating and minimizing the risk of developing type II diabetes. Through research, it has been established that the severity and symptoms of type II diabetes can be lessened with a DASH style diet. In some cases, the condition can even be reversed totally.

The foods included in the DASH diet help in improving the health of people suffering from type II diabetes. Nuts for instance improve glucose control in diabetic patients. In the same manner, diet rich in fiber content helps in slowing down the absorption of sugar which in turn balances and moderates the swings in blood sugar levels.

DASH diets contain fruits and vegetables which are rich in antioxidants. Basically, oxidants refer to free radicals distributed in the blood and cause inflammation in diabetic patients. In order to moderate the effect of these oxidants, antioxidants must be introduced so as to neutralize and stabilize them. This ultimately reduces the pain caused by tissue inflammation in diabetic patients.

Other than reducing inflammation, DASH diet helps individuals at risk of developing type II diabetes in weight loss. Excess body fat especially abdominal fat is among the biggest contributors to insulin insensitivity. Similarly, abdominal fat increases the risk of heart disease for people suffering from diabetes.

The Relationship between DASH Diet and Metabolic Syndrome

Metabolic syndrome is an umbrella term for a group of insulin-related and obesity symptoms. Commonly referred to as pre-diabetes; the metabolic syndrome often leads to type II diabetes if it not corrected in good time. The diagnostic markers of metabolic syndrome include high blood sugar levels, a large waist size, elevated HDL cholesterol, and high triglycerides. All of these symptoms are negative and can be improved if the concerned individual is placed on a DASH diet.

Having only one of these conditions does not amount to a metabolic syndrome but it must be appreciated that each of these conditions has the capacity to increase your risk of diabetes. If more than one of these symptoms occur, the chances of you developing the disease are even greater. Doctors have recommended aggressive lifestyle changes as a way of delaying the development of serious health problems.

Metabolic syndrome has its primary cause in inactivity and obesity. It is linked to a condition referred to as insulin resistance. People suffering from this condition have cells that do not respond to insulin as expected and glucose cannot enter their cells as easily. This results into glucose levels rising in your blood despite the attempt by your body to control the glucose levels. This eventually leads to diabetes.

DASH diet encourages the intake of healthy fats and fiber which are critical in lowering HDL cholesterol and levels of triglycerides. The nutrients contained in the DASH diet blend well with the fat loss action around the abdomen thus preventing reversing or significantly reducing the metabolic syndrome.

The DASH Diet and Heart Disease

People suffering from high blood pressure, metabolic syndrome and type II diabetes are vulnerable to developing heart disease. Since the DASH diet addresses all the pointers to heart disease, it in effect addresses your risk for heart disease indirectly.

There has been a misconception that the DASH diet is only for those either at risk or suffering from heart disease. The truth is, DASH diet is an excellent nutritional plan even for those who do not have these conditions. Heart disease is among the leading causes of death in America and the world as a whole. Medical practitioners have all along had an idea that a diet which is low in unhealthy fats and high in fiber could be the solution to these problems. This is what charted the waters for the research and development of the DASH diet. At the moment, this diet has gained tremendous support and endorsements thereby making it one of the most sought after heart-healthy diet.

Apart from the benefits that the DASH diet brings to the heart, it has been credited with lowering the risk of developing kidney stones, and boosts the digestive and colon health.

Fat Intake and Weight Loss

The DASH diet is very low in fat compared to the typical American diet. This also reduces the overall number of calories that the diet contributes to the body. The diet eliminates or reduces unhealthy fats which mostly come from fast foods, highly processed foods and fried foods. Since the DASH diet includes healthy fats, both saturated and unsaturated, it helps in weight loss.

Your total daily calorie intake will determine how far you go with weight loss. Fat contains about 9 calories per gram while proteins and carbohydrates contain approximately 4 calories per gram. This clearly shows that limiting your intake of fat particularly saturated fat can help you in achieving your weight loss goals faster while at the same time minimizing disease risks. According to the Institute of Medicine, fat should constitute 20 to 35 percent of your total calories and the rest filled by the other food groups.

DASH diet was formulated on the premise that unsaturated fats help in reducing the risk for heart disease. As a matter of fact, the Dietary Guidelines for Americans 2010 suggested that intake of saturated fats should be limited to 10 percent of the total calorie intake of an individual. What this means is you should consume less than 11 grams of saturated fat if you are taking a 1000 calorie diet.

Fiber and Weight Loss

The DASH diet has two main types of fibers; soluble and insoluble fibers. They play an exceptional role in helping you get rid of the body of toxins, wastes and fats as well as slowing down the absorption of sugar and fat into your bloodstream.

The slowed absorption rate helps in weight loss by reducing the amount of excess fat stored in the body and helping your body regulate and respond more efficiently to insulin. This in turn lowers the risk of metabolic syndrome.

Soluble fiber as its name suggests dissolves easily in water while the insoluble fiber does not. This is the foundational difference between these two fibers and it determines to a large extent how each of them functions within the body.

Soluble fibers attract a fair amount of water and form a gel which helps in slowing down digestion. By delaying the emptying of the stomach, these fibers make you full and help in controlling your weight.

In a similar vein, the slowed emptying of the stomach also affects the blood sugar levels and this places the soluble fibers at a strategic position in controlling diabetes. In addition to these two major functions, soluble fibers contained in the DASH diet help in fighting LDL blood cholesterol by interfering with the absorption process of dietary cholesterol.

The common sources of soluble fiber include foods such as oat cereal, oranges, apples, lentils, oat bran, flaxseeds, blueberries, celery and carrots.

Insoluble fibers on the other hand are gut-healthy because of their laxative effect and the bulk they add to diet. They help in preventing constipation since they do not dissolve in water but rather pass through the digestive tract relatively intact. This speeds up the passage of both food and waste through your gut. The source of most insoluble fibers is vegetables and whole grains.

According to research, most Americans consume about 15 grams of fiber per day on average. The

2005 Dietary Guidelines for Americans recommends an intake of about 25 grams for women under the age of 50 as well as teenage girls. For men and teenage boys, the intake was pegged at 30 to 38 grams of dietary fiber per day.

The more you increase fiber in your diet, the more you experience intestinal gas. By gradually increasing fiber, DASH diet allows the body to slowly adapt. To complement the action of soluble fiber that absorbs water in the body, you should take lots of water.

Vitamin C and Weight Loss

DASH diet is rich in vegetables and fresh fruits. These two food groups are the primary sources of minerals, essential vitamins, and antioxidants. Among these vitamins is vitamin C, also referred to as ascorbic acid. There has been a great deal of research in the recent years about vitamin C and the role it plays in weight loss specifically fat loss. Vitamin C has two main roles as far as the loss of excess fat is concerned.

Reduction in the Effects of Stress on the Body

Vitamin C helps in reducing the levels of cortisol hormone in the body. This hormone which is released into the bloodstream is the one responsible for stress. The main function of cortisol is storage of fat around the abdominal region. This storage happens as a biological insurance cover against famine.

A reduction in stress leads to a reduction in the amount of cortisol released into your system meaning, less of what you eat ends up being stored as fat in the abdomen. Prolonged reduction of cortisol gives the body an opportunity of ridding itself of abdominal fat that had accumulated before.

A Building Block for L-carnitine

L-carnitine is a compound that plays the role of transporting stored fat. The moment the signal has been sent that you no longer require the stored fat, the body metabolic processes immediately turn it back to glucose and use it as energy.

This is where L-carnitine steps in. In the body, L-carnitine is made naturally, but the process requires a good deal of Vitamin C. Ascorbic acid is soluble in water which means the body does not store much of it and as such, you need to consume it regularly.

The primary function of Vitamin C is to fight infection and rebuild body cells. After accomplishing these tasks, the remaining Vitamin C is allocated the task of generating L-carnitine. In full realization of this, the DASH diet contains the necessary quantities of Vitamin C so as to cover both the primary functions and the secondary functions of generating L-carnitine for weight loss.

Calorie Intake and Weight Loss

The conventional and mainstream approach to weight loss was based primarily on the calories in calories out formula. The logic was; the fewer the calories you take than you burn, the more promising your weight loss program will be. Despite the trust that this formula was given, recent research has revealed this is partially correct. The modern approach has that calorie reduction may lead to weight loss but not fat loss.

It is pretty common to see people who have made much progress in weight loss still appearing out of shape and flabby. The reason behind this is that a diet plan which only reduces calories results into the loss of water and lean muscle tissue instead of stored fat. This is especially the case when calories have been dramatically reduced through ambitious diet and exercise regimes.

The average American consumes about 3000 calories per day which is more than what the body requires. However, instead of pushing for a reduction of this amount, the DASH diet prescribes a caloric intake that varies from one individual to another. The factors considered in the prescription include your weight loss goals, activity level, current weight and body type. This makes the DASH diet plan a highly personalized regime that safeguards your lean muscle and gets rid of fat. It also ensures that you have sufficient nutrients to support your level of activity as well as speed up fat loss.

The DASH diet brings in a variety of healthy eating strategies thus providing a nutritional game plan for weight loss. DASH diet participants have found the plan to be realistic enough to inspire them towards their weight goals and permanent lifestyle changes.

4: How Appropriate is the DASH Diet for You

If you have a high risk of developing hypertension or you are already suffering from it, the DASH diet is a perfect solution for you. As a matter of fact, everyone needs to participate in the eating plan because it is healthy.

The increasing problem posed by obesity in the United States and elsewhere around the world tags along a related condition known as metabolic syndrome. If you are significantly overweight or your waistline is large, then chances are high that you have metabolic syndrome or are vulnerable to it.

The good news that DASH diet brings is that through its combination with exercise, it can reverse metabolic syndrome fully or partially. Even those with type II diabetes can benefit immensely from this diet plan.

Despite the rampant cases of diabetes, hypertension and metabolic syndrome, not everybody has been affected by them. For such people, the perception would be to avoid the DASH diet because it is not meant for them. However, nothing can be further from the truth; the DASH nutritional plan is also for those who are looking for a healthy way to cut weight and proactively prevent undesirable health conditions later in life.

If you are particularly considering the DASH diet for preventive and weight loss reasons, then you shall find it to be an interesting plan for your long term health. The DASH diet in its simplicity recommends that you eat foods from all the nutritional groups and guides you through the critical process of identifying and monitoring your calorie intake.

Other diets that have come before or even after the DASH diet have proposed starvation and unhealthy eating patterns as a way to force the body to shed off the extra weight. However, DASH is a healthy food–centric plan that is not only excellent but a realistic choice for many as well.

In addition to the above benefits, you will not struggle finding DASH-friendly food options while eating at a friend's house or restaurants. DASH methods to weight management are very realistic. Maintaining your ideal weight becomes a little bit easier. The diet also gives you an option to choose a sodium level that is appropriate for you.

5: How to Plan Your DASH Diet

Just as in every endeavor, good preparation is essential if you are to succeed. You should access the tools you have and whether all the supplies are in order. The goals set should also be realistic else the entire process will not be meaningful.

The DASH diet is not as complicated or difficult as it has previous been alluded. The only sacrifice that you have to make is a change in lifestyle to accommodate the new nutritional regime. To be successful on this diet, you need commitment, good planning skills and determination so you can avoid any pitfalls that may cause frustration or discouragement midstream.

Measuring Your Body Mass Index

Before you start on anything, you need to first establish your health and fitness objectives. A majority of people rely on the street or bathroom scales to know how much weight they should lose. This form of measurement is not only deceiving but also grossly inaccurate.

The starting point should be a determination of your Body Mass Index (BMI). This parameter is useful in approximating the percentage of your body weight that is fat. There are alternatives in measuring your BMI. You can have professionals help you calculate or better still purchase a body fat measurement kit. If you cannot find any of these, an online calculator and a measuring tape can do the job perfectly. The next step is to measure your weight. The best weight measurements are taken the first thing in the morning before eating or drinking anything but after urinating. You need to only wear your undergarments or nothing at all. Using a BMI assessment form, record your weight in the appropriate space provided.

There are some additional measurements that you need to take depending on your gender. For men, you will have to measure your abdomen circumference as well as your neck. Ensure that the measuring tape is in contact with your skin and does not pull too tightly. When measuring the abdomen, wrap the tape around your body just below your belly button.

In the case of women, the measurements of the circumference of the waist, neck, and hips are to be taken. The waist should be measured at the slimmest point of the torso while the hips should be measured slightly below the hip bones. The measuring tape should pass across the top portion of the buttocks. Every measurement taken should be written down one at a time on the BMI assessment form to avoid confusion.

Once all the measurements are taken, you can proceed to calculate your BMI using calculators that are available online. One of the calculators can be found at http://www.linear-software.com/online.html. To use the calculator on this link, follow the steps below in order to successfully calculate your BMI.

Enter your gender in the section provided

Input your weight and age

In the "tape measurement method" column, enter your measurements then click on the calculate button.

When you scroll below, you will find your results displayed. From the results, pick the value for your percentage body fat and record it on the BMI assessment form.

Different calculators have different interfaces but at the end of the process, they usually give you the percentage body fat metric. The reason why your body fat percentage is crucial is that it gives you a basic understanding of your current state of health.

After you start on the DASH diet, you will use the percentage body fat value to measure the extent of your progress. Recalculating your BMI instead of weighing yourself is more efficient and helps you to track your progress.

The DASH diet and the fitness workout plan helps you in gaining lean muscle mass and lose fat. The disadvantage with a weighing scale is that it cannot tell the difference between fat weight and muscle weight. Lean muscle is heavier and more compact compared to fat tissue. The scale may indicate that you have gained weight but in real sense your BMI has improved.

The Basal Metabolic Rate

Once you understand your BMI, the next crucial step is to calculate the calories your body requires to maintain its current weight. This calculation will assist you in knowing the number of calories that you should consume to lose weight at a comfortable and safe pace.

The Basal Metabolic Rate (BMR) calculation formula factors in your age, height, weight and gender. This gives you a more comprehensive and accurate answer to the number of calories that you require. Leaner body burn more calories compared to less leaner ones.

You can calculate your BMR using the following formula:

For women, the BMR equals to; 655 + (4.35 x weight in pounds) + (4.7 x height in inches) – (4.7 x age in years)

In the case of men, BMR = 66 + (6.23 x weight in pounds) + (12.7 x height in inches) – (6.8 x age in years)

Once you calculate your BMR, carefully record it on the BMI assessment form.

Your Daily Calorie Requirements

To get an accurate determination of your Daily Calorie Requirements (DCR), you should factor in your activity level. To do this, you will use the Harris Benedict Equation. The formula below shows how to determine your total daily calorie requirements using your BMR.

For people who are sedentary (little or no exercise), their DCR is BMR x 1.2.

For those who are lightly active including people who engage in sports one to three days in a week, their DCR is BMR x 1.375.

Moderately active individuals (sports three to five days in a week), their DCR equals to BMR x 1.55

Very active persons who engage in sports six to seven days in a week, their DCR equals BMR x 1.725

The last category which is said to have the highest DCR requirement consists of people who are extra active. In this category are individuals in physical jobs, sports or those who participate in intensive training. Their DCR equals BMR x 1.9

The moment you are aware of the number of calories required to maintain your weight, it becomes much easier to know the number of calories you need to eat to lose or gain weight. From scientific and laboratory measurements, one pound has been equated to 3500 calories. This means if you want to lose one pound in a week, you will have to deduct 500 calories from the sum of your daily caloric requirements. To lose two pounds, you will need to double the deduction per day.

In the case of individuals whose daily caloric requirements is already low, trying to lose weight by cutting calories may not be very practical and sustainable. Instead, it is healthier to combine decreased calorie intake and increased activity.

To start out, you can use the calorie requirements for your current activity level then subtract 500 to 1000 calories in a day. After two weeks while on your DASH to fitness plan, you should recalculate your daily calorie needs using your new activity level. This will ensure you are getting sufficient nutrition and still on track for your weight loss.

The DASH diet plan does not recommend calorie reduction below 1500 per day for women and 1800 for men.

BMI Assessment Form

Date _____

Weight _____

Neck _____

Waist _____ (Women)

Hips_____ (Women)

Abdomen _____ (Men)

Body fat % _____

BMR _____ Calories

DCR _____

In order to help you track your progress until you attain your goals, you may have to make several blank copies of the BMI assessment form.

6: Incorporating the DASH Diet into Your Lifestyle

The decision to move into a new diet plan may be slightly difficult because of the hard work and discipline required. Once you commit to incorporate the DASH diet into your lifestyle, it is important to prepare adequately for the change. To help you in this are some tips and steps to follow before starting the DASH diet.

Change in Eating Habits

Since the DASH diet will take you into a rather unconventional diet plan, it is important that you prepare beforehand by changing the way you eat. This is bound to be a challenging task and the best way to accomplish it is to eliminate all off-limits foods from your house.

This means getting rid of processed foods such as fried foods, chips and prepared snack foods. You will also have to do away with high-sodium as well as high-fat condiments such as soy sauce and salad dressings.

You have to be completely honest with yourself in this. Since you know your weaknesses better than anyone else, it is advisable you get rid of foods even if they are on the DASH diet plan. These are the foods that give you a hard time to consume in moderation.

Planning Your Menu

To achieve success with DASH diet, you have to plan your meals well in advance. You can either use the menu plans given in this book or better yet create your own customized recipes. The goal is for you to know what you will be eating during the first few weeks ahead of time. The beauty with preparing meal plans in advance is they help with shopping, elimination of unhealthy snacking and preparation for your new eating plan.

Moderating Your Taste Buds

A week before the beginning of your DASH diet, you should cut back on portion sizes, opt for fruits, remove the salt shaker from the table and skip junk foods. When focusing on these initial steps, do not worry much about your calories or any other aspects of the DASH diet. Once you start your diet plan, your body will have already adjusted to the new eating habits and the intense cravings will be gone for good.

Space Out Your Exercise Plan

Starting a new workout plan the same time as the DASH diet can be extremely overwhelming. As a matter of fact, it is considered ambitious to do this and you should not force your body to go through this kind of radical change. It is advisable you start your exercise plan either a week earlier or a week later following the beginning of your DASH diet.

You have to bear in mind that the preparation for the DASH diet is not about results but rather to provide a transition avenue to the new lifestyle. Even though a week won't be enough to make a significant difference to your health plan, it can help you ease the frustration and enhance your motivation.

Tips on How to Prepare for Success

Exercise in the mornings

When you get into a new workout routine, something always seems to get in the way of exercise. Up and until you are completely hooked onto your fitness regime and all your excuses have come to an end, it is best to exercise the first thing in the morning. You can have the liberty to change your workout schedule later on but you must wait until working out has become habitual. This usually takes about 30 days.

Reduce or eliminate salt intake

Trading your salt shaker for a salt substitute is a commendable step in preparing for the DASH diet. Even though it is impossible to completely eliminate salt from your life, planning ahead will help you to reduce significantly the quantity of salt you take. For those suffering from high blood pressure, diets that are low in sodium are recommended. There are salt substitutes and herb blends that you can use in place of salt.

Make the right choices more accessible

Healthy snacks and fresh fruits should be more visible than treats that are tempting and unhealthy. For instance, you can ward off temptation by keeping a water bottle and healthy snacks within reach. Bringing your own homemade meals to work can help you avoid the fast food lunch trap.

Drink lots of water

According to experts, you should drink at least 2 liters of water per day. This is healthy because a huge percentage of your body is water. Even if your diet is full of foods that help in digestion, you need water to make your body process work normally. Drinking lot of water also makes you feel full for longer periods and you will have more energy.

Consolidate the support of friends

The journey to healthy living requires accountability and motivation. Enlisting the support of a friend or family member when going through your diet and workouts can be such a big help. In the event you do not get anyone to walk along with you, let your friends and family know that you have embarked on a cause that is very important to you. Do not be afraid to ask for their help in fighting off the temptations that come with a new lifestyle.

Create your own customized menu

There are lots of recipes and menu plans in this book. However, these are just tools to guide you and help you in the DASH diet. They are not set in stones and as such you have the freedom to customize them. Your daily servings guide and the food list are meant to keep you on the diet without losing track.

Journalize your progress

By monitoring your progress either on a daily or weekly basis, you will have an idea of where you are headed. Jot down what you eat and the feeling you get after. These notes are important and will help you get inspired especially in moments when you hit a rough patch.

Plan for food triggers

Each one of us at some point in our lives experience triggers that make us overeat or have poor food choices. Identify your triggers and learn to figure out ways to avoid them or at least outwit them.

For instance, if you cannot watch TV without snacks, then you should get plenty of healthy snacks or alternatively eliminate watching TV for the first few weeks into the DASH diet. Once you recognize the habit inducing trigger, it becomes much easier to avoid the resulting bad habits.

Avoid stress eating

Stress eating is a common eating problem in the society today. People find it convenient to eat during stressful moments and for this reason, you need to develop an emergency plan of action before facing stressful situations.

Identify beforehand stress alleviating alternatives such as going for a short walk or spending time with a friend. Laughter and exercise release endorphins which alleviate and soothe feelings of stress. It would take you about 10 to 15 minutes to start feeling the effects and these activities will help you burn a few extra calories hence a win-win for you.

7: DASH Diet Shopping and Food Guide

The DASH diet consists of food groups that have been found through research to contain beneficial nutrients to the body. In each of these food groups are certain recommended foods which should be prioritized during shopping. Below are some of these foods categorized into groups.

Meats and Seafood

Under this category are foods such as fish particularly haddock, sardine, mackerel, and other oil fishes. Beef including roasts and lean steaks, and ground lean meat are also allowed. The DASH diet also contains chicken, eggs, game birds, ground turkey breast, lamb, and game meats. The category of meats and seafood does not allow sausages, packaged cold cats, bacon, and jerky.

Dairy Foods

This category contains blue cheese, almond milk, cow's milk, cheddar cheese, feta cheese, Greek yogurt, mozzarella cheese, provolone cheese, sour cream, soymilk, parmesan cheese, ricotta cheese, and Swiss cheese. The foods not allowed in this category include butter, full fat dairy products and cream.

Low-Glycemic Vegetables

The vegetables recommended for the DASH diet in this group include arugula, asparagus, broccoli, bell peppers, artichoke, avocadoes, brussels sprouts, cauliflower, cabbage, celery, collard greens, eggplant, cucumbers, kale, green beans, lettuce, onions, mastered greens, mushrooms, spinach, Swiss chard, turnip greens, snow peas, and summer squash.

High-Glycemic Vegetables

This includes acorn squash, carrots, butternut squash, chickpeas, English peas, sweet potatoes, tomatoes and spaghetti squash.

Corn and white potatoes should be served in very limited quantities preferably one serving per week.

Low-Glycemic Fruits

Not all fruits are included in the DASH diet. There are two main categories of fruits and these are low-glycaemic and high-glycaemic fruits. Low-glycaemic fruits include blackberries, blueberries, apples, cantaloupe, casaba melon, cranberries, guava, lemons, limes, honeydew melon, papaya, peaches, raspberries, strawberries, water melon, nectarines, and rhubarb.

High-Glycemic Fruits

This group of fruits includes mangoes, oranges, plums, pears, tangerines, figs, cherries, grapefruit, and kiwi.

Fats

The selection of fats is particularly important because a wrong step can lead you into unhealthy fats that are counterproductive to your weight loss plans. The fats allowed in this category are almonds, black walnuts, Brazil nuts, canola oil, flax seed oil, mayonnaise, olive oil, sunflower seeds and sesame seeds. The oils not allowed are peanut oil, sesame and other vegetable oils.

Grains

Whole grains are very important as sources of fiber in the body. When consumed in the right quantities, they can contribute significantly to a success of the

DASH diet and your overall weight loss. Among the grains to include in your diet are almond flour, coconut flour, wheat germ, wholegrain tortillas, whole wheat flour, whole grain pita, whole grain steel cut oats, whole grain low cab cold cereal and whole grain bread. Stay away from cornmeal, cornbread or corn muffins, flavored or instant oatmeal and sweetened cold cereals.

Seasonings and Condiments

This category comprises foods such as Caesar dressing, almond butter, coffee, dressings, flax seed oil, spices and herbs, hot sauce, iced tea, mustard peanut butter, salsa, sesame butter, peanut butter, jellies and preserves, soy sauce, tea, dill or sour pickles, spaghetti or tomato sauce, soy protein powder and vinaigrette.

Sweets

If you have a sweet tooth, the DASH diet has a special collection of sweets which are healthy and energy giving. Among these treats include dark chocolate, dried fruits, fat-free fudge pops, frozen fruit bar, ice cream, gelatin, popsicles, sorbet and pudding.

The DASH Diet Shopping Guide Tips

It must be appreciated that while on a diet, grocery shopping can be quite a challenging task. Below are a number of tips to make your shopping enjoyable and much more nutritious.

Concentrate on the edges of the store as you shop

Fresh food sections including fresh fruits and vegetables, seafood, fresh meats, fresh dairy products and poultry are normally located on the edges of the store.

Skip the danger zones

Make a deliberate effort to keep off from the aisles containing processed snacks such as cookies, chips, and crackles. Remember, getting into a DASH diet does not mean that your taste buds are completely dead as far as junk foods are concerned. The more you get these things out of your sight, the more you will get them out of your mind.

Read the labels carefully

When shopping for healthy foods, one of the things you cannot assume is the label that describes the ingredient included in the particular foodstuff.

There are some foods you cannot tell whether they are low in sodium just by simply testing them for saltiness. Read the labels on every food that you buy.

It is always advisable to make your own food right from scratch so that you can fully control the sodium content. Since this may not be possible with everyone, buying foods that are low in sugar, saturated fats and sodium is advisable. As a matter of fact, take notes of the best brands so you can easily shop without doing heavy reading.

Choose different types of produce every time you shop

One of the goals of DASH diet is to increase your intake of micronutrients and antioxidants. To achieve this, you need to vary the kinds of produce that you buy to maximize on the nutrients consumed. For instance, instead of always buying green pepper, you can change to orange or red peppers. Choose leafy and dark green vegetables and buy fruits rich in color such as mangoes, dark berries and water melons.

Choose your seafood and meat wisely

Whenever possible, purchase grass-fed, organic or pasture-raised meats and wild seafood. These foods contain lots of omega 3 fats and have less preservatives and hormones. Always be careful to choose the leanest cuts of whatever meat you are buying. After cooking, trim any visible fat to avoid unhealthy fat intake.

Choose low fat dairy

Where possible, go for low fat dairy products. The cheeses you buy should either be totally or partially non-fat. Milk is supposed to be 1 percent fat or non-fat. Yogurt on the other hand should be non-fat and contain low levels of sugar.

Your success in DASH diet will depend on the discipline that you exert while picking each of these foods.

8: The DASH Diet 14-Day Menu Planner

The secret to DASH diet success lies on the menu plans. A well designed plan will help you get accustomed to new flavors, proper portion sizes as well as combinations of healthy foods. In as much as you have the liberty to substitute the menu plans for your own recipes, you need to be mindful of calories, sodium and fat in the recipes you use.

The menu plans included in this chapter cater for a 2000-calorie diet which allows 1500 mg of sodium daily. To allow for extra helping of veggies, extra snack of fruits and an extra juice or milk beverage, the actual menus run between 1700 and 1800 calories.

If you want to adjust your calories either up or down say from 2000 to a 1600 calorie plan, you should decrease your servings of fruits or grains by one or two each. If you want to increase your calories, you should first increase your fruits and vegetables and then later on add grains.

If you feel keeping the sodium intake at a lower level is not necessary, you can be more liberal and take table salt as well as condiments such as teriyaki sauce or salad dressings. Although milk and juice are the only beverages specified in the menu plans, you can have water and sweetened coffee or tea at every meal.

Day 1 to 14 Menu Plans

The following menu plans are arranged from day 1 all the way to day 14. As stated earlier, you can customize the menus to fit into your individual preferences as long as you do not compromise on the calorie intake. Everyday has three categories of meals that are breakfast, snack, lunch, dinner and dessert.

Day 1

For breakfast, you can have two scrambled eggs, a slice of whole wheat toast with jam, a half cup cantaloupe, and 8 ounces of non-fat or 1 percent milk.

For your snack, you can have a quarter cup walnuts or raw almond. 6 ounce vanilla yogurt and a half cup blue berries.

Lunch can consist of one medium orange, a sliced chicken breast, a tablespoon of low fat salad dressing, spinach salad with tomatoes and mushrooms.

Dinner - One cup of oven roasted carrots, one whole wheat roll and south western stuffed pepper.

Dessert - One cup watermelon

Day 2

Breakfast - This can consist of a half cup cottage cheese and a pineapple/banana breakfast bowl

Snack - One medium apple, ten low sodium crackers, 4 ounces of non-fat cheese

Lunch - A slice of Swiss cheese, a half a cup of romaine lettuce, whole wheat wrap with two slices of turkey breast and mustard. You can also have one cup of low sodium chicken broth and a half cup of sliced strawberries.

Dinner - Compared to day 1, day 2 dinner is a little bit heavy with one fillet broiled fish such as cod, one cup of steamed spinach, one cup of brown rice, one half of baked sweet potato with salt substitute of margarine.

Dessert - One unsweetened and frozen fruit bar

Day 3

Breakfast - A half a cup of whole grain cereal, a quarter cup of non-fat or 1 percent milk, a half cup of strawberries and one medium banana.

Snack - One sliced tomato complete with low salad dressing and one stick string cheese

Lunch - You can have a light lunch consisting of salad with spring greens, one tablespoon low sodium dressing and red onion.

Dinner - Your dinner should consist of one broiled chicken breast with herbs, one cup of green beans with a teaspoon of olive oil or margarine and one cup of steamed quinoa with pepper and olive oil.

Dessert - You can take one medium pear

Day 4

Day 4 breakfast should consist of 6 ounce orange juice, one slice of whole wheat toast with one tablespoon jam, two egg omelet, a half cup spinach, and a quarter cup of sliced mushrooms.

Snack - A half cup of cottage cheese with a half cup peaches.

Lunch - Grilled chicken salad with one sliced chicken breast, a half cup of spinach, onions and tomatoes. You should also take one medium apple and one tablespoon vinaigrette.

Dinner - Hawaiian chicken, one cup brown rice and one sliced tomato.

Dessert - One non-fat pudding cup

Day 5

By this day, the body will have started getting accustomed to the diet and as such, you will not experience many difficulties in getting your body to accept some of the foods introduced. The meal plan is as followed:

Breakfast - 6 ounce glass of grapefruit juice and an Italian toast plate.

Snack - Your snack should consist of fruit salad with a half cup pineapple and a half cup cantaloupe. In addition, you should also have a quarter cup unsalted sunflower seeds.

Lunch - Take one cup of low sodium tomato soup made with non-fat milk, 10 low sodium crackers and one medium banana.

Dinner - A half pound steamed or boiled shrimp with cocktail sauce. One cup of sautéed kale with olive oil and salt substitute; to this add a cup of roasted carrots with olive oil and a half cup of brown rice.

Dessert - Take one large slice of honeydew melon.

Day 6

Breakfast - A half cup of sliced pears, a half whole wheat bagel with one tablespoon of jam. You can also go for tomato cheddar omelet.

Lunch - One tablespoon of low fat mayo, chicken breast sandwich with two slices of tomato, sliced onion and a half cup of lettuce. Add a medium banana to supplement your potassium needs.

Dinner - One broiled or fillet-baked salmon, one cup of steamed cauliflower with one tablespoon of olive oil or margarine as well as a half a cup sautéed onions and mushrooms. To this add 6 spears of roasted asparagus with pepper and olive oil.

Dessert - For a dessert, take one low fat fudge popsicle.

Day 7

This is the half mark of your 14 day menu plan. At this point, you should already be disciplined to take on the rest of the remaining days.

Breakfast - A half red grapefruit, a quarter cup almonds, one banana and one tablespoon coco powder with 6 ounce vanilla yogurt.

Snack - One stick non-fat or low fat string cheese and one cup honeydew melon.

Lunch - One tablespoon of balsamic vinaigrette, one slice of whole wheat toast with margarine, salad with 6 shrimp, a half cup tomato, one cup romaine lettuce and a half cup red pepper

Dinner - One cup of sautéed Swiss chard, shrimp, artichoke and scallops

Dessert - One once of square dark chocolate

Day 8

Breakfast - 6 ounce glass milk and cherry French toast.

Snack - For a snack to hold you up till lunch, you can take a half a cup of cottage cheese, a half a cup of pineapple and a quarter cup blueberries.

Lunch - 1 cup low sodium vegetable soup, a half whole wheat bagel, 1 medium apple and 1 tablespoon non-fat cream cheese.

Dinner - To crown the day, you can take a half a cup spaghetti sauce, 1 cup whole wheat, angel hair pasta, 1 tablespoon of parmesan cheese, 1 tablespoon of low fat Italian dressing, and spinach salad with onions, red peppers and mushrooms.

Dessert - You can enjoy a half a cup low fat ice cream

Day 9

Breakfast - One cup grapes, a slice of whole wheat toast with one tablespoon of margarine, two scrambled eggs and two slices of low salt turkey bacon.

Snack - Half a cup dried apricots and half a cup pumpkin seeds.

Lunch - A cup of mixed fresh berries and loaded turkey sandwich.

Dinner - 6 ounce of lean pork tenderloin, 1 cup of steamed broccoli with one tablespoon of olive oil and pepper. You can also add a half baked acorn squash with one tablespoon of margarine or olive oil and half a cup of applesauce.

Dessert - A cup of roasted fresh pineapple.

Day 10

You are on the last stretch of your 14 day meal plan. Much of the foods you take from this point up to the last day are not new anymore but a combination of several options.

Breakfast - Bacon-avocado-egg dish with 6 ounce of glass milk and a half red grape fruit.

Snack - One medium banana spread combined with one tablespoon of low salt peanut butter.

Lunch - A half a cup sautéed onions and mushrooms, one whole wheat bun, a cup of steamed green beans and 6 ounce of hamburger patty.

Dinner - 6 ounce of broiled chicken breast, one cup of steamed carrots with one tablespoon of olive oil and salt substitute, one cup of roasted zucchini and peppers.

Dessert - A cup of non-fat pudding.

Day 11

Breakfast - a half a cup 1percent milk, 1 cup of steel cut oats, 1 tablespoon honey, a quarter a cup of dried cranberries and 6 ounce glass orange juice.

Snack - One tablespoon of peanut butter, five low sodium crackers and a pear.

Lunch - A cup of low sodium minestrone, one medium mango, one whole wheat pita with a slice a mozzarella, a slice of cold roast beef, a half a cup of tomato, and one tablespoon of low sodium Italian dressing.

Dinner - Honey mustard chicken, a cup of steamed cauliflower with a tablespoon of olive oil and pepper, a cup of baked hubbard squash with one tablespoon of olive oil and nutmeg.

Dessert - One popsicle

Day 12

Breakfast - One boiled egg and blackberry quinoa bowl

Snack - Two slices of Swiss cheese, two slices of roast beef, and six whole wheat low sodium crackers.

Lunch - A half a cup blueberries, a half a cup fresh peaches and one cup of cottage cheese.

Dinner - A cup of shrimp stir-fry with 6 shrimp; a quarter cup of sprouts, carrots, onions and mushrooms. One cup brown rice

Dessert - A half a cup sorbet

Day 13

Breakfast - Half a cup of whole grain cold cereal, one medium sliced banana, a quarter a cup of one percent milk and six ounce glass orange juice.

Snack - A quarter cup walnuts and six ounce cup yogurt.

Lunch - A half a cup quinoa and shrimp kebabs.

Dinner - One cup of roasted Brussels sprouts, six ounce of lean broiled steak, one tablespoon of low sodium stick sauce, half a cup of steamed summer squash with one tablespoon of olive oil.

Dessert - One baked apple with one teaspoon honey and one teaspoon of nutmeg

Day 14

Breakfast - A half a cup low sodium granola, a quarter a cup 1 percent milk, and a half a cup sliced strawberries.

Snack - Two slices of Swiss cheese, and five low sodium crackers.

Lunch - A quarter a cup sliced onion, a quarter a cup diced tomato, one cup of grapes, one tablespoon of low sodium dressing, one wheat tortilla with three ounce sliced steak, and a quarter cup sliced onions.

Dinner - One cup frozen cheese ravioli, half a cup marinara sauce, one cup roasted butternut squash with nutmeg and one tablespoon of olive oil. You can also add one cup of steamed broccoli with one tablespoon olive oil and salt substitute.

Dessert - A cup of non-fat pudding.

Time and Event-Specific Menus

Apart from the 14 day menu plan, you can also have menus for busy workdays, weekends, and entertainment. Below are sample DASH diet menus for each of these occasions.

A Sample Menu for Busy Workdays

When busy running up and down, you may not have enough time to prepare a more comprehensive meal. This however does not mean that you should let go the discipline of healthy eating.

You can organize a simple but healthy DASH diet which fulfills all the nutritional requirements. For breakfast, you can have half a cup granola with a quarter cup 1% milk and one banana. Alternatively, you can go for peach smoothing with 6 ounces of peach yogurt, half a cup blueberries and a quarter cup non-fat milk.

When it comes to snack, you can have one banana and a quarter cup unsalted almonds. For lunch, you can take one cup Italian vegetable soup, six whole wheat crackers and two slices of provolone cheese.

Since you will be having enough time for dinner, you can prepare snapper fillet broiled with herbs and olive oil, a cup of steamed Brussels sprouts with one tablespoon of olive oil. As a source of roughage and fiber, you can have one cup of brown rice with one tablespoon margarine. To end the day healthy, you can prepare a half cup sorbet or one ounce square dark chocolate as a dessert.

Sample Menu for Weekends

Weekends are times when people relax and concentrate in family. As such, you need a meal plan that can easily fit in and give you a good time. For breakfast, you can have two scrambled eggs, half a cup cantaloupe, a slice of whole wheat toast with one tablespoon of jam.

For a snack, you can prepare one cup of fresh pineapple juice to hold you until lunch hour. One cup of low sodium tomato soup and a slice of wheat bread with a slice of mozzarella, broiled can work well for lunch.

For dinner, you can have one cup of brown rice paired with roasted winter squash and mushrooms, a thin broiled pork chop and a cup of sautéed kale. A dessert consisting of a cup of low fat pudding or a cup of fresh mango will be appropriate.

Sample Menu for Entertainment

This menu should capture the essence of the party mood without loosening on health discipline. To begin the day, you can have 6 ounce of glass orange juice, baked apple and huevos rancheros for breakfast.

A midday snack can either be low salt popcorn with garlic powder and olive oil or cucumber spears with cream cheese and smoked salmon. You can prepare a somewhat light lunch consisting of raspberry spinach salad and whole wheat roll or grilled chicken and fruit plate.

To end the day in a party mood, you can prepare peel-and-eat shrimp, grilled zucchini wedges, roasted carrots, and artichokes with one tablespoon of white wine vinaigrette for dinner. Low fat chocolate mousse or raspberry sorbet can do for a dessert.

9: DASH to Fitness Workout Plan

Apart from the DASH diet, there is the DASH to fitness workout plan which is customized for a 28-day workout period depending on your likes and dislikes as well as injuries and limitations. The DASH to fitness plan is comprehensive and includes both strength and cardio training. When planning your own individual workout program, you have two choices available; the combo plan and the alternating plan.

The alternating plan dedicates three days to cardio and another three days for strength training in alternating fashion. For instance, you may decide to do cardio on Mondays, Wednesdays and Fridays while you do strength trainings on Tuesdays, Thursdays and Saturdays. How you choose the days is totally up to you but they should be alternating. Each workout takes approximately 30 minutes.

As opposed to the alternating plan where entire days are dedicated to either strength or cardio training, the combo plan combines strength training and cardio the same day for six days each week. The only alternating option is between upper and lower body strength training. The Combo plan also comprises 30 minute workouts and is considered to be more difficult especially for beginners. It is therefore advisable to start with the alternating plan if you haven't been working out for quite some time.

After the initial workout period that is 28 days, you can change routines. Our bodies naturally become accustomed to workouts after about 21 to 30 days. Changing the intensity or type of workout can help keep your metabolism running high and this will help you avoid any plateaus. In the event you choose swimming for your cardio in the first 28 days, you may want to change to walking for the next workout period. Where you start with the alternating plan for the first workout period, you can do the combo plan for the next period.

Regardless of the workout plan you choose, you will be doing training in intervals for both cardio and strength training. Interval training is simply alternating, short harder workout segments with longer moderate workout segments. Interval training is particularly effective in building lean muscle and burning fat. It is excellent for your cardiovascular system as it revs up your metabolism and helps you get results fast.

Our bodies respond to the level of activity they are used to. If you have been sedentary for quite some time, your body will respond quickly to fast walking. For a person who has been doing exercises regularly for some time, they must walk or run in a steep incline so as to get the same results.

How to Get Started with DASH Workout Plans

The way in which DASH workout plans are designed is to accommodate every person regardless of their activity level. You do not need to have special equipment but rather a good pair of athletic shoes. However, if you are new to working out and you require instruction for specific weight training moves and stretches, you can leverage on the many websites available and DVDs that can help you.

In the event you are extremely overweight or you feel out of shape, you may begin with steady paced strength and cardio training. Do your cardio at a moderate pace from the beginning to the end of the workout and skip the cardio segments between strength training moves. After following this consistently for a month or two, you can ask your doctor whether it is safe to incorporate one of the interval training programs. In case you want to increase your workouts intensity, there are a number of ways you can achieve this. For cardio, increase the length of your intense segments and decrease the length of the moderate segments.

As an option, you can increase the incline of your treadmill, choose a much more difficulty stroke for swimming, carry small weights while walking or choose a steeper path for outdoor walking.

In strength training, you can increase the intensity of your workouts by increasing the number of reps you do or lifting slowly for increased intensity.

The Combo Workout Plans

Combo workout plans incorporate both strength training and cardio all into 30 minutes workout. You will do the same cardio workout everyday, 6 days in a week with the option of choosing from running, walking, swimming or biking plans. The lower body strength training routine and the upper body strength training regime are done on alternate days. Since both types of strength training include abdominal exercises, you can safely workout your abs without the need of a day of rest in between.

When doing combo workout plans, it is important and beneficial that you start with cardio. The goal of resistance training workout is muscle fatigue. Strength training helps in building lean muscles fast but it can be exhaustive to your muscles hence it is not advisable to strength train before heading out for run.

If you are doing strength training at home and cardio outdoors, you have no reason to worry about the downtime in between. Contrary to traditional thinking, you do not necessarily require 30 minutes of uninterrupted exercise for you to reap the benefits.

Cardio Workouts for Walking Outdoors

This is a recommended regime for cardio workouts when walking outdoors.

Take two minutes to stretch and warm up. Ensure you stretch your shoulders, neck, arms, legs and back. This helps in preparing the muscles for the exercise ahead. When you start walking, walk for 4 minutes at a moderate pace and 2 minutes at a fast pace that does not allow for any conversion. Then walk another 4 minutes at a moderate pace and 2 minutes at a fast pace. Use the last two minutes to cool down as you repeat your stretching exercises.

Cardio Workouts for Running on a Treadmill

When walking or running on a treadmill, use the first two minutes to stretch and warm up before taking the next four minutes either to walk or run at a moderate pace. Then do another two minutes of fast pace running or walking. Repeat another round of the intervals of four and two minutes. Just as in cardio workouts for walking outdoors, use the last two minutes to cool down as you repeat your stretching exercise.

Cardio Workouts for Running Outdoors

This type of workout is recommended for people who are already accustomed to running regularly. Use the first two minutes to stretch and warm up to get your systems ready. Then take four minutes to run at a moderate pace on a flat terrain and two minutes two to either run sprints or up and down stairs. Repeat these sets of four and two minutes before taking the last two minutes to cool down as you repeat the stretching exercises.

Cardio Workout for Indoor or Outdoor Cycling

Where you choose cycling as your cardio workout, prepare adequately by taking the first two minutes to stretch and warm up. Then take four minutes to cycle at low resistance or a moderate pace and two minutes to cycle at a higher resistance or a fast pace. Repeat the four and two minutes cycling sessions and afterwards take two minutes to cool down as you stretch.

Cardio Workout for Swimming

Swimming is excellent because it exercises all the major muscles of the body. By taking the first two minutes to stretch and warm up either inside or out of water, your body system will rise up to the occasion. After you are completely warmed up, use the next four minutes to swim at a moderate pace in the crawl stroke and two minutes to swim at a faster pace in the butterfly stroke. Do two reps and cool down as you engage in stretching exercises.

The Lower Body Strength Training Routine

This training requires only one minute for warm up through stretching. Then do five lunges with your right leg and another five with your left leg until you complete 20 lunges total. Take one minute to run in place, do jumping jacks or jump rope. Do ten squats and then take one minute to jump rope or run in place before doing 20 hamstring lifts.

With one minute in between, do twenty modified crunches where you lift until your shoulders leave the floor and do twenty leg lifts or what is known as reverse crunches. After every session of the lower body training routine, cool down by repeating the stretching exercises.

Upper Body Strength Training Routine

Begin this session by taking a minute to warm up as you stretch. Then do twenty pushups, twenty seated chair dips, twenty alternating crunches also known as scissor or oblique crunches. In between each of these workouts, take one minute to jump rope, run in place or do jumping jacks. At the end of the session, take a minute to cool down.

Alternating Workout Plans

Once you go through the combo plan successfully, the alternating workout plan should not pose any difficulty because the same steps and moves are used. The only difference is that you are combining workouts and doing them in alternating days. In three days per week, you will do cardio workouts while in the remaining days you will do combined strength training workout.

Cardio

This workout takes 30 minutes and you simply choose your preferred method of doing cardio from the combo plans. Double the number of segments except for the warm up and cool down times.

Strength Training Routine

This routine involves 2 minutes of warming up by stretching followed by 20 front lunges, 10 squats, 20 hamstring lifts also known as toe raises, 20 leg lifts, 20 modified crunches, 20 alternating crunches, 20 pushups and 20 seated chair dips. These are done with a minute in between for jump rope or jumping jacks. The last two minutes are for the body to cool down.

10: The DASH Diet Cookbook Recipes

In the previous chapters, we have seen the various meals that are recommended in the DASH diet plan. While some of these meals are familiar and easy to prepare, others may be a little bit strange hence the need for guidelines on how to prepare them. This chapter is dedicated to DASH diet recipes ranging from breakfast all the way to dinner.

Breakfast Recipes

The breakfast recipes explained include cranberry almond spread, toasted egg sandwich, tropical fruit and yogurt bowl, mushroom and Swiss omelet, spring asparagus brunch plate, pumpkin pie for breakfast among others.

Cranberry Almond Spread

Cranberries are foods rich in vitamin C while the almonds provide a crunch and extra nutrition which makes this spread delicious. You can spoon it over yogurt or spread it on a bagel for dessert and breakfast respectively. This is how you prepare it:

Ingredients:

One cup fresh cranberries

A half a cup unsweetened orange juice

A pinch of sugar

One tablespoon of cornstarch

One tablespoon of water

A half a cup slivered almonds

One cup vanilla extract

Procedure:

Chop the cranberries carefully and add them to a non-stick saucepan and pour the orange juice. Warm the mixture gently over medium heat and add sugar to taste. Mix the cornstarch and water in a cup until the mixture smoothens. Then turn the heat to low before pouring in the cornstarch mixture as you stir. Raise the heat to medium high to allow the mixture to simmer until it thickens. Remove the pan from the heat and stir in the vanilla and almonds. You can cover and chill the cranberry almond spread and store it up in a refrigerator to last you for two weeks. This spread can make one and a half cup.

Toasted Egg Sandwich

This is a light breakfast rich in fiber and proteins. Instead of the red pepper that is included among the ingredients, you can use onion, mushroom or tomato.

Ingredients:

A slice of whole wheat bread

Canola oil spray

Two ounce slice turkey bacon

One large egg

A thin slice of chopped red bell pepper

A thin slice of low fat jack cheese

Fresh ground black pepper

Procedure:

Coat a non-sticky skillet with canola oil and place over medium heat and toast the slice of bread on one side in the skillet. When it has turned light brown, set it aside on a plate with the toasted side facing up. Add the turkey bacon to the skillet and ensure that it cooks on both sides. Then remove it and set it on top of the toasted bread. Break the egg into the skillet and coax it around using a spatula so that it measures approximately the size and shape the slice of toast. When it barely sets, remove it from the pan and place it gently on top of the sandwich.

Then transfer the sandwich into the skillet and top it with cheese and the sliced pepper. Then cover the pan with a lid and turn the heat to medium low. When the cheese has melted, transfer the entire sandwich back to the plate and sprinkle it lightly with the fresh ground black pepper.

Tropical Fruit and Yogurt Bowl

Yogurt and fruit is a combination that makes an excellent breakfast that can also be served as a snack for the afternoon. This mixture has essential enzymes, antioxidants and vitamin C.

Ingredients:

A half a cup diced fresh mango

A half a cup diced fresh pineapple

A half a cup diced fresh papaya

A cup of low fat and unsweetened yogurt

Fresh mint

Honey, low fat granola and cinnamon where desired

Procedure

Combine the yogurt and fruits in a bowl and stir gently. Transfer the mixture into two individual bowls. Where preferred, you can top each serving with a dash of cinnamon or a small drizzle of honey. Garnish with a couple of fresh mint leaves.

Mushroom and Swiss Omelet

The extra egg whites provide protein to the omelet. You can add diced tomato or olives where desired.

Ingredients:

Two eggs and two egg whites

One tablespoon of non-fat milk

Canon oil spray

A half a cup sliced fresh mushrooms

One ounce of low fat Swiss cheese either shredded or cubed

One diced green onion

Fresh ground black pepper

As an option, you can have red salsa or non-fat sour cream

The Procedure

Warm the omelet pan over a medium low heat for about a minute. As the pan is heating, whisk the eggs lightly with the milk but do not over mix the eggs. Coat the omelet pan with canola oil spray and allow it to warm for another 15 seconds. Add the mushrooms to the pan and let them cook for a minute while stirring once or twice. Pour the eggs to the pan but do not stir them.

Once you notice the edges beginning to firm up a bit, use a heat proof rubber spatula to slide down around the edges and gently lift to let the liquid eggs on top flow under the edges to the bottom of the pan. This is particularly excellent where you lift the edges of the omelet in four or five spots around the edge of the pan. Arrange the green onion and the cheese across half of the omelet. Sprinkle the freshly ground black pepper.

Continue cooking the omelet and slide a larger flat spatula under one side of the omelet and gently fold it over the other half to form a half circle. Slide the folded omelet over to the center of the pan. Use the spatula to press lightly on the top of the omelet so as to coax any remaining liquid out into the pan.

Cover the pan with a lid and remove it from the heat. You can allow the omelet to sit for about a minute as you finish setting the eggs and then slide the omelet into a plate and serve. You can top it up with non-fat sour cream or red salsa for extra flavor.

Lunch Recipes

The DASH diet comes with lots of meal options for lunch. Among these recipes include South Western salmon, Rosemary chicken, Dijon pork chops, shrimp kebabs, New York turkey melts, honey mustard chicken, and loaded turkey sandwich among others.

Southwestern Salmon

For the best flavor, you can use freshly ground pepper. Also, the spice that is used on the salmon can be used on chicken or pork.

Ingredients:

Six ounce salmon fillet

One Anaheim chilly

One medium tomato

Canola oil spray

A pinch of freshly ground black pepper

A pinch of chili powder

A pinch of cumin

A pinch of onion powder

A half cup of unsweetened orange juice

Procedure

Rinse the salmon carefully and then part it with a paper towel. Remove the seeds, stem and veins of the chili and slice it into a half an inch rinse. Cut the tomato into wedges and warm the skillet over medium heat and coat it with canola oil spray. Lay the salmon fillet at the middle of the pan and arrange the tomato and chili around it. Combine a pinch of black pepper, cumin, onion powder and chili powder into a small dish. Sprinkle the spice blend on the salmon and vegetables and cover the pan.

Cook for about six minutes and then add the orange juice. Cover the pan again and turn off the heat leaving the pan on the banner. After three minutes, check the salmon if it is opaque and no longer translucent. It is ready to serve.

Rosemary Chicken

This is easier and quicker to make and can be served cold or hot. You can also decide to take it chilled and sliced with coleslaw or sweet potato salad.

Ingredients:

Canola oil spray

Twelve ounce skinless chicken breast

Four medium tomatoes

Black pepper

A tablespoon of red wine vinegar

Two sprigs fresh Rosemary and a half a cup of dry white wine

Procedure

Coat an eight inch glass baking dish lightly with canola oil spray. Arrange the chicken in the dish and dust fresh ground black pepper over it. Cut the tomatoes into quarters and carefully arrange them around the chicken. Sprinkle the vinegar over the tomatoes and tuck the rosemary next to the chicken. Pour the white wine into the dish and cover with a foil. Bake the contents for about 35 minutes. Slice the chicken breast and toss it with the rest of the ingredients ready for serving.

Shrimp Kebabs

Kebabs make one of the most attractive and tasty lunches. Nutrition-wise, kebabs are almost fat free, high in iron and a good source of protein.

Ingredients:

Fifteen to twenty raw shrimps or prawns

A half fresh pineapple, peeled and its top removed

One red bell pepper

A small red onion

A tablespoon of rice vinegar

Two tablespoons of olive oil

One tablespoon of fresh chopped oregano

Six cherry tomatoes

Cajun seasoning

Procedure

Peel and rinse the shrimp on paper towels. Cut the pineapples into sixteen chunks measuring about one and half inches each. Remove the stem and seeds from the bell pepper and cut it into small bite-sized pieces. Cut the onion into small pieces and mix the vinegar or oregano and oil into a small bowl. Thread the pineapple, shrimp and vegetables onto skewers and carefully lay them on the baking sheet. Brush the oil mixture on the kebabs and coat each piece well.

You can now preheat the grill and brush the kebabs with the oil mixture again. Before you grill, dust lightly with Cajun seasoning. The grilling is to take about five minutes on each side or until the prawns or shrimps are browned on the outside.

The New York Turkey Melts

This recipe will help you satisfy a deli sandwich craving. You can add a variety of cheeses and vegetables to enhance the texture and flavor of the meal.

Ingredients:

Two tablespoons of fat free cream cheese

Four slices of low sodium rye bread

A teaspoon of horseradish

Six ounces of sliced roast turkey breast

A half small thinly sliced cucumber

A half small thinly sliced red onion

Two thin slices provolone

Canola oil spray

Procedure

Spread two bread slices with horseradish and cream cheese. Layer the turkey, onion, cucumber, and provolone. Top each layering with a slice of bread. Coat your pan with canola oil spray and slowly toast the sandwiches over a medium heat until browned.

Honey Mustard Chicken

This dish is easier to prepare hence making it an excellent choice for busy weeknights. You can even make some extra for lunch the following day.

Ingredients:

A tablespoon of olive oil

Four skinless and boneless chicken thighs

A half a cup slivered almonds

A half a cup low sodium vegetable broth

A half a cup dry white wine

Two tablespoons of yellow mustard

One tablespoon of honey

Freshly ground black pepper

Procedure

Heat a non-stick skillet over a medium heat and then add olive oil. Gently add the chicken to the pan and give it time to brown on all sides. Blend the broth, almonds, mustard, wine and honey in a food processor until smooth. You can season with black pepper to taste. When the chicken has browned, pour over it the honey-mustard mixture and cover the pan with a lid. With the heat turned to low, simmer gently for around fifteen minutes.

Snacks and Appetizers

There are various dishes you can prepare as snacks and appetizers that will not jeopardize your DASH diet regime. Some of these snacks include garlic basil shrimp, stuffed mushrooms, watermelon smoothes, avocado cheese melts and many others.

Garlic Basil Shrimp

There is an option to make this on skewers. Ensure you soak the skewers in water for a period of about thirty minutes so as to prevent them from burning.

Ingredients:

One tablespoon of melted and unsalted butter

Fifteen to twenty raw shrimps

Twelve large basil leaves

Two tablespoons of mixed garlic

A half a cup of dry white wine

Procedure

Pre-heat the broiler and then add butter to a broiler-safe pan. Peel and rinse the shrimps before wrapping them with a basil leaf. Add garlic and spread it around the pan then add the wrapped shrimp. Broil for about a minute, turn the shrimp over and add the white one. Broil again until the shrimp is ready; this should take about four minutes.

Stuffed Mushrooms

When preparing stuffed mushrooms, beware of parmesan cheese because it is high in sodium. Low fat shredded mozzarella can be a perfect substitute because of its low sodium content.

Ingredients:

Twelve large fresh mushrooms

A quarter a cup grated parmesan cheese

A half a cup panko breadcrumbs

Two tablespoons of finely chopped green onions

A quarter cup of non-fat sour cream

Procedure

Preheat the broiler and remove the stems from the mushrooms. Chop the stems finely and combine mushrooms, cheese, breadcrumbs and green onions in a bowl. Stir the sour cream and mix well. Then stuff the caps of the mushrooms with the mixture and place them on a broiler pan for broiling until they become tender and brown.

Dinner Recipes

There are various options in the DASH diet when it comes to dinner. Some of these options include tender lemon chicken, Italian beef stew, broccoli rice bake, and spicy Southwest chili.

Italian Beef Stew

Ingredients:

One small chopped yellow onion

A half pound extra lean ground beef

One tablespoon of mixed garlic

One cup of tomato juice

One tablespoon of Italian seasoning

One tablespoon of minced garlic

One cup of tomato juice

One cup of sliced mushrooms

A cup of black coffee

Three quarters of a cup dry red wine

A cup of orzo

Procedure

Put a large non-stick stock pot over a medium heat and brown the beef with the onion inside it. Then add the garlic, Italian seasoning and mushrooms while stirring for about two to three minutes. Add the coffee, tomato juice and wine. Add the orzo when the liquid starts simmering. Stir gently and simmer for about 15 minutes on low heat.

Conclusion

The DASH diet is a roadmap to a healthier lifestyle. It is flexible and designed to enable you make necessary changes as swiftly as possible. You can also modify the program as to fit your personal needs as your fitness and health improves. The DASH diet is not another quick fix to health improvement. Instead, it is backed by scientific research and provides a new way of living and a productive commitment to better health.

The DASH diet methods are built on proven and sound nutritional advice. They help in reducing sodium to lower hypertension and its associated risks, it increases fiber which steadies the blood sugar levels, reduced blood pressure and assist in weight loss. The diet also minimizes Trans fat and saturated fat to increase heart health, raise good cholesterol, lower bad cholesterol and aid in weight loss. The healthy fats in your body get a boost through the intake of seeds, nuts, avocado and fish among other omega 3 rich foods.

The recipes contained in this book are just but the beginning.

To reap the most from the DASH diet, you have to be consistent and explorative. Remember the DASH diet journey is for your own benefit and as such, you are to take charge.